Homeopathic Gemstone Therapy Presented

Dr Víctor Denis Purcell and Victor Denis Purcell

Published by Victor Denis Purcell, 2024.

While every precaution has been taken in the preparation of this book, the publisher assumes no responsibility for errors or omissions, or for damages resulting from the use of the information contained herein.

HOMEOPATHIC GEMSTONE THERAPY PRESENTED

First edition. August 29, 2024.

ISBN: 979-8227727329

Written by Dr Víctor Denis Purcell and Victor Denis Purcell.

"Homeopathic Gemstone Therapy Presented"

Homeopathic Medicine Defined:

Homeopathic medicine represents a deeply holistic and profoundly natural approach to healing, one that views the individual as an integrated whole rather than a mere collection of symptoms. The origins of homeopathy trace back to the late 18th century, where the inquisitive mind of Dr. Samuel Hahnemann, a German physician disillusioned with the harsh medical practices of his era, sought a gentler path to healing. Through rigorous experimentation and a deep understanding of medicinal substances, Hahnemann formulated the foundational principles of homeopathy, most notably the Law of Similars—often encapsulated in the phrase "like cures like." This principle posits that a substance capable of producing certain symptoms in a healthy individual can, when administered in highly diluted form, treat those same symptoms in someone who is unwell. Hahnemann's pioneering work laid the groundwork for a system of medicine that prizes gentle, individualized treatment, a system that has since found resonance across the globe, embraced by millions who seek a more harmonious path to health.

The preparation of homeopathic remedies is a meticulous process, distinguished by the method of serial dilution and succussion—a vigorous shaking that is believed to enhance the energetic properties of the original substance. Known as potentization, this process involves repeatedly diluting the active ingredient in a mixture, often of water or alcohol, and then shaking it forcefully. The result is a remedy that, paradoxically, contains only minute traces, or sometimes none at all, of the original substance, yet is considered to possess profound healing potential. This method of preparation aligns with the core homeopathic belief that healing can occur on an energetic level, transcending the material presence of the medicinal substance itself.

The sources of homeopathic remedies are vast and varied, drawing from the rich resources of the natural world, including plants, minerals, and animal derivatives. The selection of a remedy is not merely a matter of addressing physical symptoms but involves a comprehensive assessment of the patient's physical, emotional, and psychological state. This individualized approach is a hallmark of homeopathy, reflecting its core philosophy that each person's path to healing is unique. Homeopathic practitioners, therefore, dedicate significant time to understanding the totality of their patient's condition, seeking not just to alleviate symptoms, but to uncover and address the deeper, underlying causes of illness.

One of the most remarkable aspects of homeopathy is its capacity to stimulate the body's intrinsic healing mechanisms. Rather than merely suppressing symptoms, as is often the case with conventional treatments, homeopathy seeks to engage the body's own restorative processes, encouraging a return to balance and health. This gentle, non-invasive approach holds particular appeal for those who wish to avoid the side effects commonly associated with pharmaceutical drugs. In aligning with the body's natural rhythms, homeopathy offers a path to healing that is not only safe but deeply respectful of the body's innate wisdom and capacity for self-regulation.

The philosophy of homeopathy is intimately connected with the concept of vitalism, which posits that a vital force or energy animates the body and governs its overall health. According to this perspective, disease arises from an imbalance or disturbance in this vital force, and the role of the homeopathic remedy is to gently restore harmony. This view resonates with those drawn to holistic and alternative forms of medicine, as it acknowledges the interconnectedness of body, mind, and spirit in the healing process. Homeopathy thus broadens the understanding of health, viewing it not merely as the absence of disease, but as a dynamic state of balance and well-being.

Despite its enduring appeal and the countless testimonies of healing attributed to it, homeopathy has long been met with skepticism, particularly from the scientific community. The highly diluted nature of its remedies and the challenges in explaining its mechanisms within the framework of conventional science have led to ongoing debate. Yet, homeopathy has persisted and flourished, a testament to its profound impact on those who have experienced its healing touch. For many, the personal and anecdotal evidence of its efficacy outweighs the lack of scientific validation, making homeopathy a cherished and enduring form of medicine.

Homeopathy's contribution to global health is both significant and far-reaching, particularly in regions where conventional medical resources are scarce. Its accessibility, affordability, and ease of administration make it an invaluable tool in public health, particularly in the developing world. Additionally, in more affluent societies, where there is a growing interest in natural and holistic approaches, homeopathy is experiencing a resurgence. More individuals are seeking alternatives to the impersonal and often side-effect-laden treatments offered by conventional medicine, finding in homeopathy a compassionate and patient-centered approach to health care.

In the complex landscape of modern healthcare, homeopathy stands as a beacon of ancient wisdom, offering a deeply compassionate and individualized approach to healing. It honors the uniqueness of each person's journey to wellness, respecting the body's natural processes and trusting in its capacity to heal itself. In a world that often prioritizes quick fixes and symptomatic relief, homeopathy reminds us of the importance of addressing the whole person, of seeking balance, and of harnessing the gentle yet profound power of nature to restore health and harmony.

Disclaimer

The information presented in this book is for educational and entertainment purposes only. It is not intended to serve as medical advice or to replace professional healthcare services. If you are experiencing any discomfort, illness, or have health concerns, please consult a qualified healthcare professional or physician. Always seek the advice of your physician or other qualified health providers with any questions you may have regarding a medical condition.

Presentation of Popular Healing Homeopathic Gemstones

In this section, we explore a selection of the most popular gemstones known for their profound healing benefits. These gemstones have been cherished across cultures and times for their ability to support physical, emotional, and spiritual well-being. Whether you are new to gemstone healing or a seasoned practitioner, these stones are essential additions to your collection, offering a wide range of therapeutic effects. The material is presented in similar fashion to traditional homeopathic medicines that are found in homeopathy Materia Medica.

Amethyst Homeopathic Remedy: A New Path to Holistic Healing

Amethyst, now introduced as a homeopathic remedy, represents an exciting new development in the integration of traditional gemstone healing with the principles of homeopathy. This remedy, derived from the natural amethyst stone, is revered for its deep and holistic effects on mental, emotional, psychological, and physical health, offering a comprehensive approach to well-being that resonates with both ancient wisdom and modern therapeutic practices.

Mentally, amethyst as a homeopathic remedy is renowned for its ability to clear the mind of negative thoughts, confusion, and mental fog. It acts as a stabilizing force, particularly beneficial for those who find themselves overwhelmed by scattered thoughts or difficulty in maintaining focus. This remedy enhances cognitive function, allowing for clearer thinking, better memory retention, and a more efficient processing of information. By promoting mental clarity, amethyst helps individuals make well-considered decisions, navigate complex situations with ease, and reduce the mental stress that often accompanies a busy and demanding life. Its influence extends to soothing an overactive mind, bringing about a sense of mental calm and peace that can be invaluable in high-pressure environments or during periods of intense intellectual activity.

Emotionally, the amethyst homeopathic remedy serves as a powerful ally for those experiencing emotional imbalance or distress. It has traditionally been used to alleviate symptoms associated with anxiety, depression, and emotional instability, offering a gentle yet effective approach to emotional healing. The calming energy of amethyst helps to pacify intense emotions, providing relief from overwhelming feelings such as fear, anger, or profound sadness. It fosters emotional balance by helping individuals reconnect with their inner selves, promoting self-awareness, and encouraging the expression of true emotions in a constructive and healthy manner. This remedy is particularly beneficial during times of emotional upheaval or transition, offering support and stability as one navigates through challenging emotional landscapes.

Psychologically, the amethyst remedy is deeply connected to the enhancement of spiritual awareness and the development of higher consciousness. It is especially useful for those on a spiritual journey, as it aids in opening the third eye and crown chakras, which are essential for accessing deeper states of meditation and spiritual insight. Amethyst homeopathic remedy assists in the cultivation of intuition and the enhancement of psychic abilities, making it a valuable tool for individuals seeking to expand their spiritual horizons or those who work within intuitive or healing professions. Additionally, it provides a protective shield against negative energies and psychic attacks, safeguarding psychological well-being and ensuring that one's spiritual practice remains pure and untainted by external influences.

Physically, the amethyst homeopathic remedy has a broad range of applications, rooted in its historical use as a powerful healing stone. It is known to strengthen the immune system, providing the body with the resilience needed to fend off illnesses and recover more quickly from physical ailments. Amethyst is also effective in reducing pain, particularly that associated with tension headaches, migraines, and other stress-related conditions. Its influence on circulation is noteworthy, as it helps to improve blood flow and oxygenation throughout the body, contributing to overall vitality and well-being. This remedy is frequently used to address sleep disorders, particularly insomnia, by promoting a state of relaxation that facilitates restful and restorative sleep. Furthermore, amethyst supports the body's natural detoxification processes, aiding in the elimination of toxins and contributing to the maintenance of optimal physical health.

The historical significance of amethyst as a healing stone further enhances its value as a homeopathic remedy. In ancient civilizations, amethyst was prized for its supposed ability to prevent intoxication, protect the mind, and promote clarity of thought. Today, these properties are harnessed through homeopathic preparation, allowing this age-old wisdom to be applied to contemporary health concerns. The amethyst homeopathic remedy stands as a bridge between the past and the present, bringing the timeless healing qualities of this gemstone into the realm of modern medicine. It offers a unique and versatile solution for those seeking holistic healing, providing support across a wide range of physical, mental, emotional, and psychological conditions.

As a new addition to the world of homeopathy, the amethyst remedy embodies the integration of ancient traditions with modern therapeutic approaches. Its ability to address mental clarity, emotional soothing, psychological protection, and physical healing makes it a multifaceted remedy that can be utilized in various contexts, from everyday wellness to more specific therapeutic applications. Amethyst homeopathic remedy is a testament to the enduring power of natural medicine, offering a gentle yet profound approach to achieving balance, peace, and holistic well-being in today's fast-paced world. Whether used as a preventative measure or as part of a broader treatment plan, amethyst continues to shine as a beacon of healing, guiding individuals towards a more harmonious and fulfilled life.

Aquamarine: A Calming Force for Holistic Well-Being

Aquamarine is a gemstone of remarkable beauty and potency, known for its profound healing properties that have been cherished across cultures for centuries. This serene and captivating stone integrates ancient wisdom with a holistic approach to well-being, offering a comprehensive pathway to balance and tranquility in all aspects of life. As a symbol of the sea, aquamarine embodies the essence of water—fluid, purifying, and calming—making it a powerful ally for mental, emotional, psychological, and physical health.

Mentally, aquamarine is celebrated for its soothing influence on the mind, providing clarity and focus in the midst of life's challenges. In today's fast-paced world, where mental overload and stress are common, aquamarine offers a much-needed respite. This gemstone is particularly effective for individuals who find themselves overwhelmed by the demands of daily life, helping to quiet racing thoughts and promote a sense of inner peace. Aquamarine clears mental clutter, allowing for a more organized and peaceful thought process, which is essential for decision-making, problem-solving, and creative thinking. For those engaged in intellectually demanding tasks or facing complex challenges, aquamarine serves as a stabilizing force, enhancing cognitive function and improving concentration. The cooling energy of aquamarine not only dispels anger and irritability but also fosters a deeper understanding and acceptance of situations, allowing individuals to approach life's difficulties with a calm and rational mindset.

Emotionally, aquamarine is known for its gentle yet powerful healing properties. It has traditionally been used to alleviate emotional imbalances, particularly those related to fear, anxiety, and unresolved trauma. In times of emotional turbulence, aquamarine acts as a comforting presence, helping individuals navigate their emotions with greater ease and grace. The soothing energy of aquamarine helps dissolve emotional blockages, enabling the release of pent-up emotions and facilitating the healing process. This gemstone is especially beneficial for those who struggle with deep-seated fears or anxieties, offering a sense of security and calm that can be transformative. Aquamarine encourages emotional resilience, empowering individuals to maintain emotional stability even in the face of adversity. By fostering an environment of tranquility, aquamarine promotes healthy emotional expression and strengthens the connection with one's inner self, leading to a more balanced and fulfilling emotional life.

Psychologically, aquamarine is revered for its ability to enhance communication and self-expression. This gemstone is particularly effective for individuals who struggle with expressing their thoughts and feelings or who experience difficulty in communicating effectively with others. Aquamarine works by opening the throat chakra, which is the energy center associated with communication and self-expression. By doing so, it facilitates clear and honest communication, helping individuals to overcome the fear of speaking or shyness that may hinder their ability to express themselves fully. Aquamarine also fosters courage, particularly in situations where one needs to stand up for themselves, assert their boundaries, or speak their truth. On a deeper psychological level, aquamarine supports the release of old, limiting beliefs and patterns that may be holding individuals back from reaching their full potential. This gemstone is a powerful tool for those on a path of self-discovery, offering clarity and insight into one's true nature, desires, and life purpose. As a result, aquamarine helps to cultivate greater self-awareness, self-confidence, and personal growth, paving the way for a more authentic and empowered existence.

Physically, aquamarine is highly regarded for its ability to support the body's natural healing processes. This gemstone has a cooling and calming effect on the body, making it particularly useful for conditions associated with inflammation, fever, or heat-related symptoms.

Aquamarine has traditionally been used to support respiratory health, offering relief from symptoms such as sore throat, laryngitis, or bronchitis. Its soothing properties also extend to the eyes, where it can alleviate eye strain, reduce puffiness, and support overall eye health. Aquamarine's benefits are not limited to the respiratory system; its cooling and calming energy is also effective for the skin, where it can reduce redness, irritation, or inflammation. Additionally, aquamarine is believed to strengthen the immune system, enhancing the body's ability to fend off illness and recover more quickly from physical ailments. It also plays a crucial role in the detoxification process, aiding in the elimination of toxins and contributing to overall physical well-being. By supporting the body's natural defenses and promoting balance, aquamarine helps to maintain optimal health and vitality.

Historically, aquamarine has been revered for its calming and protective qualities, making it a treasured gemstone across various cultures and traditions. In ancient times, aquamarine was considered a gift from the sea and was believed to be the stone of mermaids, offering protection to sailors and ensuring safe voyages. It was often used as an amulet or talisman, worn by those seeking to invoke the powers of the sea for protection, healing, and spiritual insight. Aquamarine has long been associated with the water element, symbolizing purity, tranquility, and emotional clarity. These attributes are harnessed in modern times to allow individuals to benefit from aquamarine's timeless healing properties. Whether used in meditation, healing rituals, or as part of a daily wellness routine, aquamarine continues to serve as a bridge between ancient traditions and contemporary therapeutic practices, offering a versatile and effective approach to holistic healing.

Aquamarine brings the gentle yet powerful energy of this beloved gemstone into the realm of modern wellness, making it a valuable tool for those seeking to achieve balance, tranquility, and holistic well-being. Its ability to calm the mind, soothe the emotions, enhance communication, and support physical health makes aquamarine a multifaceted remedy that can be used in a variety of contexts, from everyday wellness to more specific therapeutic needs. As a testament to the enduring power of natural healing, aquamarine offers a pathway to peace and harmony, guiding individuals towards a more balanced, peaceful, and fulfilling life. Whether used as a preventative measure or as part of a broader wellness plan, aquamarine continues to shine as a beacon of healing, offering a timeless source of support and inspiration for those on their journey to well-being.

Ruby: A Vital Force for Holistic Well-Being.

Ruby is a gemstone of unparalleled vitality and brilliance, revered for its potent healing properties that have been cherished across cultures for millennia. This radiant and dynamic stone seamlessly integrates ancient wisdom with a holistic approach to well-being, offering a comprehensive pathway to strength, energy, and emotional warmth. As a symbol of life force, passion, and courage, ruby embodies the essence of fire—vibrant, energizing, and purifying—making it an indispensable ally for mental, emotional, psychological, and physical health.

Mentally, ruby is celebrated for its invigorating influence on the mind, providing clarity, motivation, and a zest for life. In an era where mental fatigue, indecision, and lack of focus are prevalent, ruby offers a revitalizing boost that sharpens the intellect and enhances mental acuity. This gemstone is particularly effective for individuals who struggle with lethargy, procrastination, or a sense of mental stagnation, providing the necessary spark to reignite one's passion and drive. Ruby stimulates the mind, helping to dispel doubts and confusion, allowing for clear, decisive, and strategic thinking. Its energizing properties encourage a proactive and confident approach to challenges, empowering individuals to overcome obstacles and achieve their goals with determination. For those engaged in creative or strategic endeavors, ruby serves as a catalyst for innovation, problem-solving, and dynamic thinking, fostering a positive and ambitious mindset. The warming energy of ruby not only combats mental exhaustion but also ignites a passion for learning and growth, inspiring individuals to pursue their aspirations with renewed enthusiasm and vigor.

Emotionally, ruby is known for its unparalleled ability to ignite and sustain passion, love, and enthusiasm for life. It has traditionally been used to enhance emotional resilience and foster a deep sense of joy, fulfillment, and connection with one's desires. In times of emotional turmoil, apathy, or heartbreak, ruby acts as a powerful motivator, rekindling the inner fire and restoring a sense of purpose, vitality, and emotional balance. The energizing influence of ruby helps to dissolve emotional blockages, enabling individuals to experience and express their emotions more fully and authentically. This gemstone is especially beneficial for those who have lost touch with their desires, who feel disconnected from their emotions, or who are seeking to reignite the passion within their relationships. Ruby offers a pathway to emotional awakening, renewal, and transformation, empowering individuals to embrace their emotions with courage and authenticity. By fostering an environment of warmth, vitality, and emotional clarity, ruby promotes a deeper connection with one's passions, desires, and purpose, leading to a more vibrant, joyful, and fulfilling emotional life.

Psychologically, ruby is revered for its profound ability to enhance self-confidence, personal power, and leadership qualities. This gemstone is particularly effective for individuals who struggle with feelings of inadequacy, self-doubt, fear of failure, or reluctance to take charge of their lives. Ruby works by stimulating the root and heart chakras, which are closely associated with personal power, grounding, emotional well-being, and the courage to pursue one's goals. By doing so, ruby fosters a strong sense of self-worth, personal empowerment, and the confidence to take bold actions in the pursuit of one's dreams and aspirations. Ruby also enhances the ability to set and maintain healthy boundaries, enabling individuals to assert their needs, desires, and intentions in a balanced, respectful, and effective manner. On a deeper psychological level, ruby supports the release of old patterns of fear, shame, guilt, and self-limitation that may be holding individuals back from embracing their true potential. This gemstone is a powerful tool for those on a journey of self-discovery, offering clarity, insight, and the courage to live authentically, passionately, and purposefully. As a result, ruby helps to cultivate greater self-awareness, personal empowerment, and the determination to face life's challenges with resilience and confidence.

Physically, ruby is highly regarded for its ability to support the body's vitality, endurance, and overall health. This gemstone has a warming, energizing, and invigorating effect on the body, making it particularly useful for conditions associated with low energy, fatigue, poor circulation, or cold extremities. Ruby has traditionally been used to support cardiovascular health, as it is believed to strengthen the heart, improve blood flow, and enhance the body's ability to maintain optimal circulation. Its invigorating properties also extend to the reproductive system, where ruby is used to enhance fertility, sexual vitality, and overall reproductive health. Ruby's benefits are not limited to the circulatory and reproductive systems; its warming energy is also effective in boosting the body's natural defenses, enhancing the immune system's ability to fend off illness and promote rapid recovery from physical ailments. Additionally, ruby is believed to play a crucial role in the detoxification process, aiding in the elimination of toxins, purifying the blood, and contributing to overall physical well-being and vitality. By enhancing the body's natural strength, vitality, and resilience, ruby helps to maintain optimal health, energy levels, and physical endurance, making it an indispensable ally for those seeking to achieve peak physical condition.

Historically, ruby has been revered for its protective, energizing, and transformative qualities, making it one of the most treasured gemstones across various cultures, traditions, and spiritual practices. In ancient times, ruby was considered the stone of kings, warriors, and leaders, believed to confer strength, courage, wisdom, and protection in battle. It was often worn as a talisman or embedded in armor to safeguard against harm, enhance the wearer's physical and mental strength, and invoke the warrior spirit. Ruby has long been associated with the fire element, symbolizing passion, strength, the life force, and the eternal flame of the heart. These attributes are harnessed in modern times to allow individuals to benefit from ruby's timeless healing properties.

Whether used in meditation, healing rituals, or as part of a daily wellness routine, ruby continues to serve as a bridge between ancient traditions and contemporary therapeutic practices, offering a versatile, dynamic, and effective approach to holistic healing and well-being.

Ruby brings the dynamic, powerful, and transformative energy of this beloved gemstone into the realm of modern wellness, making it an invaluable tool for those seeking to achieve strength, vitality, and holistic well-being. Its unparalleled ability to energize the mind, ignite the emotions, enhance personal power, and support physical health makes ruby a multifaceted remedy that can be used in a variety of contexts, from everyday wellness to more specific therapeutic needs. As a testament to the enduring power of natural healing, ruby offers a pathway to vibrant, passionate, and empowered living, guiding individuals towards a more resilient, fulfilled, and harmonious life. Whether used as a preventative measure, a source of inspiration, or as part of a broader wellness plan, ruby continues to shine as a beacon of energy, strength, and transformation, offering a timeless source of support and empowerment for those on their journey to holistic well-being.

Lapis Lazuli: A Stone of Wisdom and Spiritual Insight

Lapis Lazuli is a gemstone of profound depth and timeless beauty, revered across cultures for its powerful healing and spiritual properties. This deep blue stone, often flecked with gold, seamlessly integrates ancient wisdom with a holistic approach to well-being, offering a comprehensive pathway to inner truth, clarity, and spiritual enlightenment. As a symbol of wisdom, truth, and the higher mind, Lapis Lazuli embodies the essence of intellectual and spiritual clarity, making it a powerful ally for mental, emotional, psychological, and physical health.

Mentally, Lapis Lazuli is celebrated for its ability to enhance intellectual abilities and stimulate the desire for knowledge and understanding. In a world where information is abundant but true wisdom is scarce, Lapis Lazuli offers a guiding light that helps to illuminate the mind, fostering critical thinking, clarity, and the pursuit of truth. This gemstone is particularly effective for individuals who seek to deepen their intellectual pursuits, offering a clear and focused mind that is receptive to new ideas and insights. Lapis Lazuli helps to dispel mental confusion, enabling one to see situations more clearly and to make well-informed decisions. Its energizing properties encourage a quest for knowledge and a deeper understanding of the self and the world around us. For those engaged in intellectual work or spiritual studies, Lapis Lazuli serves as a powerful tool for enhancing concentration, memory, and the ability to grasp complex concepts, fostering a sharp and insightful mindset. The calming yet stimulating energy of Lapis Lazuli not only clears mental blockages but also opens the mind to higher truths and deeper understanding, empowering individuals to approach life's challenges with wisdom and discernment.

Emotionally, Lapis Lazuli is known for its ability to harmonize emotions and promote deep emotional healing. It has traditionally been used to help individuals connect with their inner truth, enabling them to express their emotions and thoughts authentically and with clarity. In times of emotional turmoil, confusion, or suppression, Lapis Lazuli acts as a catalyst for self-expression, helping individuals to articulate their feelings and needs with confidence and honesty. The harmonizing influence of Lapis Lazuli helps to balance the emotions, fostering a state of calm and equilibrium. This gemstone is especially beneficial for those who struggle with emotional repression, fear of judgment, or difficulty in communicating their true feelings. Lapis Lazuli encourages emotional honesty and self-awareness, empowering individuals to embrace their true selves and to communicate their emotions openly and effectively. By fostering an environment of emotional clarity and authenticity, Lapis Lazuli promotes healthy emotional expression and a deeper connection with one's inner wisdom and truth.

Psychologically, Lapis Lazuli is revered for its ability to enhance self-awareness, intuition, and spiritual insight. This gemstone is particularly effective for individuals who seek to deepen their spiritual practice or who are on a journey of self-discovery. Lapis Lazuli works by stimulating the third eye and throat chakras, which are closely associated with intuition, spiritual insight, and self-expression. By doing so, Lapis Lazuli fosters a strong connection to the higher self and the spiritual realms, enabling individuals to access their inner wisdom and to perceive the deeper truths of existence. Lapis Lazuli also enhances the ability to see beyond the surface, promoting a deeper understanding of oneself and others. On a deeper psychological level, Lapis Lazuli supports the release of limiting beliefs and patterns that may be hindering spiritual growth and self-awareness. This gemstone is a powerful tool for those who seek to cultivate greater self-awareness, personal empowerment, and spiritual insight, offering clarity, guidance, and the courage to live authentically and in alignment with one's true purpose. As a result, Lapis Lazuli helps to cultivate a deep sense of inner peace, spiritual wisdom, and the confidence to navigate life's challenges with grace and understanding.

Physically, Lapis Lazuli is highly regarded for its ability to support the body's overall health and well-being, particularly in areas related to the throat, respiratory system, and immune function. This gemstone has a cooling and soothing effect on the body, making it particularly useful for conditions associated with inflammation, throat irritation, or respiratory issues. Lapis Lazuli has traditionally been used to support throat health, alleviate sore throats, and reduce symptoms of laryngitis or bronchitis. Its calming properties also extend to the nervous system, where it can help to alleviate stress-related conditions such as headaches, tension, or anxiety. Lapis Lazuli's benefits are not limited to the respiratory and nervous systems; its cooling energy is also effective in supporting the immune system, enhancing the body's ability to fend off illness and promote overall health. Additionally, Lapis Lazuli is believed to support the detoxification process, aiding in the elimination of toxins and contributing to overall physical vitality and well-being. By enhancing the body's natural defenses and promoting balance, Lapis Lazuli helps to maintain optimal health and resilience.

Historically, Lapis Lazuli has been revered for its spiritual and intellectual qualities, making it one of the most treasured gemstones across various cultures, traditions, and spiritual practices. In ancient Egypt, Lapis Lazuli was considered the stone of the gods, believed to provide access to divine wisdom and spiritual insight. It was often used in amulets, jewelry, and sacred artifacts to enhance spiritual connection and to invoke protection. Lapis Lazuli has long been associated with the element of air, symbolizing intellect, clarity, and the higher mind. These attributes are harnessed in modern times to allow individuals to benefit from Lapis Lazuli's timeless healing properties. Whether used in meditation, healing rituals, or as part of a daily wellness routine, Lapis Lazuli continues to serve as a bridge between ancient traditions and contemporary therapeutic practices, offering a versatile and effective approach to holistic healing and spiritual well-being.

Lapis Lazuli brings the profound, wise, and spiritually enlightening energy of this beloved gemstone into the realm of modern wellness, making it an invaluable tool for those seeking to achieve clarity, spiritual insight, and holistic well-being. Its unparalleled ability to stimulate the intellect, harmonize the emotions, enhance spiritual insight, and support physical health makes Lapis Lazuli a multifaceted remedy that can be used in a variety of contexts, from everyday wellness to more specific therapeutic needs. As a testament to the enduring power of natural healing, Lapis Lazuli offers a pathway to enlightened, empowered, and harmonious living, guiding individuals towards a more fulfilled, spiritually attuned, and harmonious life. Whether used as a preventative measure, a source of spiritual guidance, or as part of a broader wellness plan, Lapis Lazuli continues to shine as a beacon of wisdom, spiritual clarity, and insight, offering a timeless source of support and enlightenment for those on their journey to holistic well-being.

Moonstone: A Beacon of Intuition and Emotional Balance

Moonstone is a gemstone of ethereal beauty and profound emotional resonance, revered across cultures for its powerful healing and intuitive properties. This captivating stone, with its delicate shimmer and iridescent hues, seamlessly integrates ancient wisdom with a holistic approach to well-being, offering a comprehensive pathway to emotional balance, intuition, and inner harmony. As a symbol of the moon's calming and nurturing energy, Moonstone embodies the essence of emotional equilibrium and spiritual insight, making it a powerful ally for mental, emotional, psychological, and physical health.

Mentally, Moonstone is celebrated for its ability to calm the mind and enhance intuitive thinking. In a world where logical reasoning often overshadows emotional intelligence, Moonstone offers a gentle reminder of the importance of balance between the mind and heart. This gemstone is particularly effective for individuals who struggle with overthinking, anxiety, or stress, providing a soothing balm that quiets the mind and encourages a more intuitive approach to problem-solving. Moonstone helps to dispel mental confusion and self-doubt, allowing for clearer thinking and greater trust in one's inner guidance. Its nurturing energy encourages a receptive and open-minded attitude, making it easier to tune into one's intuition and to make decisions that are aligned with one's true desires. For those engaged in creative or reflective pursuits, Moonstone serves as a muse, enhancing imagination, inspiration, and the ability to see beyond the ordinary. The calming yet illuminating energy of Moonstone not only clears mental blockages but also opens the mind to the subtle wisdom of the inner self, empowering individuals to navigate life's challenges with grace and clarity.

Emotionally, Moonstone is known for its unparalleled ability to balance and soothe the emotions, offering deep emotional healing and support. It has traditionally been used to help individuals connect with their emotions in a healthy and constructive way, fostering emotional awareness and resilience. In times of emotional upheaval, instability, or overwhelm, Moonstone acts as a comforting presence, helping individuals to process and release negative emotions such as fear, anger, or sadness. The nurturing influence of Moonstone helps to stabilize mood swings, reduce emotional volatility, and promote a sense of inner peace and calm. This gemstone is especially beneficial for those who are sensitive to the emotional energies of others, as it provides a protective and grounding force that shields against emotional overwhelm. Moonstone encourages emotional healing and self-compassion, empowering individuals to embrace their emotions with kindness and understanding. By fostering an environment of emotional balance and harmony, Moonstone promotes healthy emotional expression and a deeper connection with one's inner self, leading to a more peaceful and fulfilling emotional life.

Psychologically, Moonstone is revered for its ability to enhance intuition, spiritual insight, and self-awareness. This gemstone is particularly effective for individuals who seek to deepen their connection with their inner wisdom or who are on a journey of spiritual growth. Moonstone works by stimulating the third eye and crown chakras, which are closely associated with intuition, spiritual awareness, and the higher self. By doing so, Moonstone fosters a strong connection to the subconscious mind and the spiritual realms, enabling individuals to access their inner guidance and to perceive the deeper truths of existence. Moonstone also enhances the ability to recognize and trust one's intuitive feelings, promoting a deeper understanding of oneself and the world around them. On a deeper psychological level, Moonstone supports the release of old emotional patterns and beliefs that may be hindering personal growth and self-awareness. This gemstone is a powerful tool for those who seek to cultivate greater self-awareness, spiritual insight, and personal empowerment, offering clarity, guidance, and the courage to live authentically and in alignment with one's true purpose. As a result, Moonstone helps to cultivate a deep sense of inner peace, spiritual wisdom, and the confidence to navigate life's challenges with grace and understanding.

Physically, Moonstone is highly regarded for its ability to support the body's overall health and well-being, particularly in areas related to the reproductive system, hormonal balance, and emotional health. This gemstone has a cooling and soothing effect on the body, making it particularly useful for conditions associated with stress, anxiety, or hormonal imbalances. Moonstone has traditionally been used to support reproductive health, alleviate menstrual discomfort, and balance hormones, making it especially beneficial for women. Its calming properties also extend to the digestive system, where it can help to alleviate stress-related digestive issues such as bloating, nausea, or indigestion. Moonstone's benefits are not limited to the reproductive and digestive systems; its cooling energy is also effective in promoting restful sleep, reducing symptoms of insomnia, and enhancing overall emotional well-being. Additionally, Moonstone is believed to support the body's natural rhythms, such as the menstrual cycle and the sleep-wake cycle, contributing to overall physical vitality and harmony. By enhancing the body's natural balance and promoting emotional resilience, Moonstone helps to maintain optimal health and well-being.

Historically, Moonstone has been revered for its intuitive and emotional qualities, making it one of the most treasured gemstones across various cultures, traditions, and spiritual practices. In ancient Rome, Moonstone was believed to be formed from the light of the moon, and it was often used as a talisman for protection and guidance during travel. In Hindu mythology, Moonstone is associated with the divine feminine and is believed to bring good fortune and enhance fertility. Moonstone has long been associated with the water element, symbolizing the ebb and flow of emotions and the cycles of life. These attributes are harnessed in modern times to allow individuals to benefit from Moonstone's timeless healing properties. Whether used in meditation, healing rituals, or as part of a daily wellness routine, Moonstone continues to serve as a bridge between ancient traditions and contemporary therapeutic practices, offering a versatile and effective approach to holistic healing and emotional well-being.

Moonstone brings the gentle, nurturing, and intuitively enlightening energy of this beloved gemstone into the realm of modern wellness, making it an invaluable tool for those seeking to achieve emotional balance, spiritual insight, and holistic well-being. Its unparalleled ability to calm the mind, balance the emotions, enhance intuition, and support physical health makes Moonstone a multifaceted remedy that can be used in a variety of contexts, from everyday wellness to more specific therapeutic needs. As a testament to the enduring power of natural healing, Moonstone offers a pathway to peaceful, balanced, and intuitively guided living, guiding individuals towards a more harmonious, fulfilled, and spiritually attuned life. Whether used as a preventative measure, a source of emotional support, or as part of a broader wellness plan, Moonstone continues to shine as a beacon of emotional healing, intuition, and inner harmony, offering a timeless source of support and guidance for those on their journey to holistic well-being.

Peridot: A Stone of Renewal and Positive Energy

Peridot is a gemstone of vibrant energy and rejuvenation, revered across cultures for its powerful healing properties and its ability to inspire positive change. This bright green stone, with its rich and invigorating hues, seamlessly integrates ancient wisdom with a holistic approach to well-being, offering a comprehensive pathway to renewal, protection, and emotional healing. As a symbol of growth, transformation, and abundance, Peridot embodies the essence of renewal and the nurturing power of the earth, making it a powerful ally for mental, emotional, psychological, and physical health.

Mentally, Peridot is celebrated for its ability to clear the mind of negative thoughts and promote a positive outlook. In a world where stress, anxiety, and pessimism can often cloud one's thinking, Peridot offers a refreshing burst of clarity and optimism. This gemstone is particularly effective for individuals who struggle with self-doubt, fear, or negative thought patterns, providing a mental reset that encourages a more positive and constructive mindset. Peridot helps to dispel mental confusion and self-limiting beliefs, allowing for clearer thinking and a greater sense of self-confidence. Its energizing properties encourage a proactive approach to life's challenges, making it easier to overcome obstacles and to see opportunities where there once were limitations. For those engaged in creative or problem-solving activities, Peridot serves as a catalyst for inspiration, innovation, and the ability to think outside the box. The uplifting energy of Peridot not only clears mental blockages but also opens the mind to new possibilities, empowering individuals to approach life with renewed hope and enthusiasm.

Emotionally, Peridot is known for its ability to heal and protect the heart, offering deep emotional support and resilience. It has traditionally been used to help individuals release old emotional wounds, forgive themselves and others, and move forward with a sense of peace and closure. In times of emotional turmoil, heartbreak, or grief, Peridot acts as a soothing balm, helping individuals to process and release negative emotions such as anger, resentment, or bitterness. The protective influence of Peridot helps to shield the heart from further emotional harm, creating a safe space for healing and renewal. This gemstone is especially beneficial for those who are recovering from emotional trauma or who are seeking to rebuild their self-esteem and trust in others. Peridot encourages emotional healing and self-compassion, empowering individuals to let go of past hurts and to embrace a brighter, more positive future. By fostering an environment of emotional protection and renewal, Peridot promotes healthy emotional expression and a deeper connection with one's inner strength and wisdom, leading to a more balanced and fulfilling emotional life.

Psychologically, Peridot is revered for its ability to enhance self-worth, personal empowerment, and resilience. This gemstone is particularly effective for individuals who struggle with feelings of inadequacy, low self-esteem, or a lack of motivation. Peridot works by stimulating the solar plexus and heart chakras, which are closely associated with personal power, self-confidence, and emotional well-being. By doing so, Peridot fosters a strong sense of self-worth and the confidence to pursue one's goals and dreams with determination and courage. Peridot also enhances the ability to set and maintain healthy boundaries, making it easier to protect oneself from negative influences and to prioritize one's well-being. On a deeper psychological level, Peridot supports the release of old patterns of fear, guilt, or shame that may be holding individuals back from achieving their true potential. This gemstone is a powerful tool for those on a journey of self-discovery and personal growth, offering clarity, guidance, and the strength to live authentically and in alignment with one's true purpose. As a result, Peridot helps to cultivate greater self-awareness, personal empowerment, and the resilience to face life's challenges with confidence and grace.

Physically, Peridot is highly regarded for its ability to support the body's overall health, vitality, and recovery. This gemstone has a detoxifying and revitalizing effect on the body, making it particularly useful for conditions associated with toxicity, sluggishness, or fatigue. Peridot has traditionally been used to support the health of the liver and digestive system, as it is believed to enhance the body's ability to detoxify and to metabolize nutrients effectively. Its revitalizing properties also extend to the skin, where Peridot is used to promote a clear and radiant complexion. Peridot's benefits are not limited to the digestive and integumentary systems; its energizing energy is also effective in boosting the body's natural defenses, enhancing the immune system's ability to fend off illness and promote recovery from physical ailments. Additionally, Peridot is believed to support the body's ability to regenerate and renew, making it a valuable tool for those recovering from illness or injury. By enhancing the body's natural vitality and promoting balance, Peridot helps to maintain optimal health and energy levels, contributing to overall physical well-being.

Historically, Peridot has been revered for its protective, rejuvenating, and transformative qualities, making it a treasured gemstone across various cultures, traditions, and spiritual practices. In ancient Egypt, Peridot was known as the "gem of the sun" and was believed to have the power to ward off evil spirits and to bring prosperity and abundance. It was often worn as an amulet or embedded in jewelry to invoke protection, renewal, and the nurturing energy of the earth. Peridot has long been associated with the element of earth, symbolizing growth, healing, and the cycles of life. These attributes are harnessed in modern times to allow individuals to benefit from Peridot's timeless healing properties. Whether used in meditation, healing rituals, or as part of a daily wellness routine, Peridot continues to serve as a bridge between ancient traditions and contemporary therapeutic practices, offering a versatile and effective approach to holistic healing and well-being.

Peridot brings the vibrant, protective, and rejuvenating energy of this beloved gemstone into the realm of modern wellness, making it an invaluable tool for those seeking to achieve renewal, emotional healing, and holistic well-being. Its unparalleled ability to clear the mind, protect the heart, enhance self-worth, and support physical health makes Peridot a multifaceted remedy that can be used in a variety of contexts, from everyday wellness to more specific therapeutic needs. As a testament to the enduring power of natural healing, Peridot offers a pathway to positive, empowered, and rejuvenated living, guiding individuals towards a more resilient, fulfilled, and harmonious life. Whether used as a preventative measure, a source of emotional support, or as part of a broader wellness plan, Peridot continues to shine as a beacon of renewal, protection, and positive energy, offering a timeless source of support and transformation for those on their journey to holistic well-being.

Rose Quartz: A Stone of Unconditional Love and Emotional Healing

Rose Quartz is a gemstone of gentle beauty and profound emotional depth, revered across cultures for its powerful healing properties and its ability to open the heart to unconditional love. This soft pink stone, with its soothing and nurturing energy, seamlessly integrates ancient wisdom with a holistic approach to well-being, offering a comprehensive pathway to emotional healing, self-love, and compassion. As a symbol of love, peace, and harmony, Rose Quartz embodies the essence of unconditional love and emotional balance, making it a powerful ally for mental, emotional, psychological, and physical health.

Mentally, Rose Quartz is celebrated for its ability to calm the mind and promote a loving and compassionate perspective. In a world where stress, anxiety, and emotional turmoil can often cloud one's thinking, Rose Quartz offers a soothing presence that encourages a more gentle and understanding approach to life's challenges. This gemstone is particularly effective for individuals who struggle with negative self-talk, fear of rejection, or feelings of unworthiness, providing a mental reset that encourages self-compassion and positive thinking. Rose Quartz helps to dispel mental tension and emotional stress, allowing for clearer thinking and a greater sense of inner peace. Its nurturing energy encourages a mindset of acceptance and love, making it easier to approach oneself and others with kindness and empathy. For those engaged in healing work, counseling, or seeking emotional clarity, Rose Quartz serves as a comforting guide, enhancing emotional insight and the ability to navigate life's complexities with a loving heart. The gentle energy of Rose Quartz not only calms mental turbulence but also opens the mind to the healing power of love, empowering individuals to cultivate a more compassionate and harmonious outlook on life.

Emotionally, Rose Quartz is known for its unparalleled ability to heal the heart and restore emotional balance, offering deep emotional support and comfort. It has traditionally been used to help individuals open their hearts to love, both for themselves and others, fostering emotional healing and forgiveness. In times of emotional pain, grief, or heartache, Rose Quartz acts as a gentle balm, helping individuals to process and release negative emotions such as sadness, anger, or fear. The nurturing influence of Rose Quartz helps to heal emotional wounds and to restore a sense of trust and openness in relationships. This gemstone is especially beneficial for those who have experienced loss, betrayal, or emotional trauma, offering a pathway to emotional renewal and the courage to love again. Rose Quartz encourages self-love and self-acceptance, empowering individuals to embrace their true selves and to cultivate healthy, loving relationships. Its influence can also extend to family dynamics, where it can help to ease tensions and promote understanding. By fostering an environment of emotional healing and compassion, Rose Quartz promotes healthy emotional expression and a deeper connection with one's inner self, leading to a more peaceful and fulfilling emotional life.

Psychologically, Rose Quartz is revered for its ability to enhance self-love, emotional resilience, and inner peace. This gemstone is particularly effective for individuals who struggle with feelings of inadequacy, self-criticism, or emotional instability. Rose Quartz works by stimulating the heart chakra, which is closely associated with love, compassion, and emotional well-being. By doing so, Rose Quartz fosters a strong sense of self-worth and the confidence to embrace one's emotions with understanding and compassion. Rose Quartz also enhances the ability to forgive, both oneself and others, making it easier to let go of past hurts and to move forward with an open heart. On a deeper psychological level, Rose Quartz supports the release of old patterns of fear, guilt, or resentment that may be hindering emotional growth and self-awareness. This gemstone is a powerful tool for those on a journey of emotional healing and personal growth, offering clarity, guidance, and the strength to live authentically and with love. Rose Quartz's ability to soothe emotional turmoil makes it a valuable companion during times of change or transition, providing stability and reassurance. As a result, Rose Quartz helps to cultivate greater self-awareness, emotional balance, and the resilience to face life's challenges with grace and compassion.

Physically, Rose Quartz is highly regarded for its ability to support the body's overall health, particularly in areas related to the heart, circulation, and emotional well-being. This gemstone has a calming and soothing effect on the body, making it particularly useful for conditions associated with stress, tension, or emotional strain. Rose Quartz has traditionally been used to support heart health, improve circulation, and promote a sense of physical and emotional well-being. Its calming properties also extend to the skin, where Rose Quartz is used to promote a clear and radiant complexion, reduce signs of aging, and soothe irritated or inflamed skin. Rose Quartz's benefits are not limited to the heart and skin; its soothing energy is also effective in supporting restful sleep, reducing symptoms of insomnia, and enhancing overall emotional and physical relaxation. Additionally, Rose Quartz is believed to support the body's ability to heal from emotional trauma and to promote a sense of peace and harmony within the physical body. Its gentle nature makes it an ideal gemstone for those recovering from illness or those seeking to maintain emotional and physical balance. By enhancing the body's natural balance and promoting emotional resilience, Rose Quartz helps to maintain optimal health and well-being.

Historically, Rose Quartz has been revered for its loving and healing qualities, making it one of the most treasured gemstones across various cultures, traditions, and spiritual practices. In ancient Egypt, Rose Quartz was believed to have anti-aging properties and was used in facial masks and healing rituals to promote beauty and love. In Greek mythology, Rose Quartz is said to have been created by the goddess

Aphrodite, symbolizing love and beauty. Rose Quartz has long been associated with the element of water, symbolizing purity, emotional healing, and the flow of love. These attributes are harnessed in modern times to allow individuals to benefit from Rose Quartz's timeless healing properties. Whether used in meditation, healing rituals, or as part of a daily wellness routine, Rose Quartz continues to serve as a bridge between ancient traditions and contemporary therapeutic practices, offering a versatile and effective approach to holistic healing and emotional well-being.

Rose Quartz brings the gentle, loving, and emotionally healing energy of this beloved gemstone into the realm of modern wellness, making it an invaluable tool for those seeking to achieve emotional balance, self-love, and holistic well-being. Its unparalleled ability to calm the mind, heal the heart, enhance self-love, and support physical health makes Rose Quartz a multifaceted remedy that can be used in a variety of contexts, from everyday wellness to more specific therapeutic needs. As a testament to the enduring power of natural healing, Rose Quartz offers a pathway to loving, compassionate, and emotionally balanced living, guiding individuals towards a more harmonious, fulfilled, and heart-centered life. Whether used as a preventative measure, a source of emotional support, or as part of a broader wellness plan, Rose Quartz continues to shine as a beacon of love, healing, and inner peace, offering a timeless source of support and transformation for those on their journey to holistic well-being.

Topaz: A Stone of Manifestation and Clarity

Topaz is a gemstone of luminous beauty and powerful energy, revered across cultures for its transformative properties and its ability to manifest intentions into reality. This vibrant stone, which can range in color from golden yellow to deep blue, seamlessly integrates ancient wisdom with a holistic approach to well-being, offering a comprehensive pathway to clarity, purpose, and personal empowerment. As a symbol of truth, abundance, and manifestation, Topaz embodies the essence of clarity and intention, making it a powerful ally for mental, emotional, psychological, and physical health.

Mentally, Topaz is celebrated for its ability to clear the mind and enhance focus, helping individuals to align their thoughts with their goals. In a world where distractions and mental clutter can often impede progress, Topaz offers a beacon of clarity that illuminates the path forward. This gemstone is particularly effective for individuals who struggle with indecision, procrastination, or a lack of motivation, providing a mental reset that encourages clear thinking and purposeful action. Topaz helps to dispel confusion and mental fog, allowing for sharper focus and the ability to make well-informed decisions. Its energizing properties encourage a proactive approach to life's challenges, making it easier to set goals and follow through with determination and confidence. For those engaged in creative or strategic endeavors, Topaz serves as a catalyst for innovation, problem-solving, and the ability to bring ideas to fruition. The illuminating energy of Topaz not only clears mental blockages but also aligns the mind with the power of intention, empowering individuals to manifest their desires and achieve their fullest potential.

Emotionally, Topaz is known for its ability to uplift the spirit and inspire a sense of joy and abundance. It has traditionally been used to help individuals cultivate a positive outlook, release negative emotions, and embrace the beauty of life. In times of emotional stagnation, doubt, or fear, Topaz acts as a radiant force that dispels darkness and brings light to the heart. The uplifting influence of Topaz helps to dissolve emotional blockages, enabling individuals to release feelings of sadness, frustration, or hopelessness. This gemstone is especially beneficial for those who are seeking to attract positivity and abundance into their lives, offering a pathway to emotional renewal and the courage to pursue happiness. Topaz encourages emotional resilience and optimism, empowering individuals to embrace life's challenges with grace and confidence. By fostering an environment of emotional clarity and abundance, Topaz promotes healthy emotional expression and a deeper connection with one's inner joy and purpose, leading to a more vibrant and fulfilling emotional life. Its influence extends to personal relationships as well, where it can help to strengthen bonds, enhance communication, and bring about greater understanding and harmony between individuals.

Psychologically, Topaz is revered for its ability to enhance self-confidence, personal power, and the ability to manifest one's desires. This gemstone is particularly effective for individuals who struggle with feelings of self-doubt, insecurity, or a lack of direction. Topaz works by stimulating the solar plexus and third eye chakras, which are closely associated with personal power, intuition, and clarity of vision. By doing so, Topaz fosters a strong sense of self-worth and the confidence to pursue one's goals with determination and enthusiasm. Topaz also enhances the ability to visualize and manifest intentions, making it easier to attract opportunities and to create the life one desires. On a deeper psychological level, Topaz supports the release of old patterns of fear, scarcity, or limitation that may be holding individuals back from achieving their true potential. This gemstone is a powerful tool for those on a journey of personal growth and manifestation, offering clarity, guidance, and the strength to live authentically and with purpose. As a result, Topaz helps to cultivate greater self-awareness, personal empowerment, and the resilience to manifest one's dreams into reality. Its ability to help individuals align their inner goals with their outer actions makes Topaz an invaluable tool for those seeking to make lasting, positive changes in their lives.

Physically, Topaz is highly regarded for its ability to support the body's overall health, vitality, and energy. This gemstone has an invigorating and regenerative effect on the body, making it particularly useful for conditions associated with fatigue, low energy, or sluggishness. Topaz has traditionally been used to support the health of the digestive system, as it is believed to enhance the body's ability to absorb nutrients and to metabolize energy efficiently. Its energizing properties also extend to the nervous system, where Topaz is used to promote mental clarity, reduce stress, and enhance overall cognitive function. Topaz's benefits are not limited to the digestive and nervous systems; its revitalizing energy is also effective in boosting the immune system, enhancing the body's natural defenses, and promoting rapid recovery from physical ailments. Additionally, Topaz is believed to support the body's ability to regenerate tissues and to promote overall physical resilience. This gemstone is also thought to aid in detoxification, helping to cleanse the body of impurities and promoting a sense of physical renewal. By enhancing the body's natural vitality and promoting balance, Topaz helps to maintain optimal health and energy levels, contributing to overall physical well-being.

Historically, Topaz has been revered for its manifestation and protective qualities, making it a treasured gemstone across various cultures, traditions, and spiritual practices. In ancient Greece, Topaz was believed to enhance strength and to provide protection in battle, often worn as an amulet by warriors and leaders. In Renaissance Europe, Topaz was associated with wealth and was believed to attract abundance and success to its wearer. In Hindu culture, Topaz is revered as a symbol of divine favor and spiritual enlightenment, often worn to enhance wisdom and to connect with higher realms. Topaz has long been associated with the element of fire, symbolizing transformation, clarity, and the power of intention. These attributes are harnessed in modern times to allow individuals to benefit from Topaz's timeless healing properties. Whether used in meditation, healing rituals, or as part of a daily wellness routine, Topaz continues to serve as a bridge between ancient traditions and contemporary therapeutic practices, offering a versatile and effective approach to holistic healing and personal empowerment.

Topaz brings the radiant, clarifying, and empowering energy of this beloved gemstone into the realm of modern wellness, making it an invaluable tool for those seeking to achieve clarity, manifestation, and holistic well-being. Its unparalleled ability to clear the mind, uplift the spirit, enhance personal power, and support physical health makes Topaz a multifaceted remedy that can be used in a variety of contexts, from everyday wellness to more specific therapeutic needs. As a testament to the enduring power of natural healing, Topaz offers a pathway to clear, empowered, and purpose-driven living, guiding individuals towards a more fulfilled, abundant, and harmonious life. Whether used as a preventative measure, a source of inspiration, or as part of a broader wellness plan, Topaz continues to shine as a beacon of manifestation, clarity, and inner strength, offering a timeless source of support and transformation for those on their journey to holistic well-being.

Turquoise: A Stone of Protection and Spiritual Grounding

Turquoise is a gemstone of ancient heritage and profound spiritual significance, revered across cultures for its protective properties and its ability to bring peace and balance. This captivating stone, with its distinct blue-green hue, seamlessly integrates ancient wisdom with a holistic approach to well-being, offering a comprehensive pathway to spiritual grounding, emotional healing, and protection. As a symbol of wisdom, tranquility, and protection, Turquoise embodies the essence of spiritual balance and inner peace, making it a powerful ally for mental, emotional, psychological, and physical health.

Mentally, Turquoise is celebrated for its ability to bring clarity and calm to the mind, helping to alleviate stress, anxiety, and mental exhaustion. In a world where the mind is often overburdened by worries and fears, Turquoise provides a soothing balm that encourages mental serenity and a clearer perspective. This gemstone is particularly effective for individuals who struggle with overthinking, worry, or a sense of mental instability, providing a calming influence that helps to quiet the mind and restore a sense of peace. Turquoise helps to dispel negative thought patterns and mental confusion, allowing for a more balanced and centered approach to life's challenges. Its grounding properties encourage a mindful approach to daily life, making it easier to navigate complex situations with wisdom and calmness. For those engaged in meditation, spiritual practices, or simply seeking mental clarity, Turquoise serves as a guide, enhancing focus, intuition, and the ability to connect with higher states of consciousness. The tranquil energy of Turquoise not only clears mental blockages but also aligns the mind with spiritual wisdom, empowering individuals to approach life with a sense of peace and spiritual clarity.

Emotionally, Turquoise is known for its powerful ability to heal emotional wounds and to bring balance to the heart and emotions. It has traditionally been used to help individuals release old emotional patterns, heal from past traumas, and restore a sense of emotional equilibrium. In times of emotional upheaval, heartache, or grief, Turquoise acts as a gentle protector, helping individuals to process and release negative emotions such as fear, sadness, or anger. The nurturing influence of Turquoise helps to create a safe and supportive space for emotional healing, allowing individuals to rebuild their emotional strength and resilience. This gemstone is especially beneficial for those who feel emotionally drained or overwhelmed, offering a pathway to emotional renewal and the courage to embrace life with a renewed sense of hope and joy. Turquoise encourages emotional honesty and self-expression, empowering individuals to communicate their feelings with clarity and compassion. By fostering an environment of emotional healing and balance, Turquoise promotes healthy emotional expression and a deeper connection with one's inner self, leading to a more peaceful and harmonious emotional life.

Psychologically, Turquoise is revered for its ability to enhance spiritual awareness, inner wisdom, and protection. This gemstone is particularly effective for individuals who seek to deepen their spiritual practice or who are on a journey of self-discovery and spiritual growth. Turquoise works by stimulating the throat and third eye chakras, which are closely associated with communication, intuition, and spiritual insight. By doing so, Turquoise fosters a strong connection to the higher self and the spiritual realms, enabling individuals to access their inner wisdom and to perceive the deeper truths of existence. Turquoise also enhances the ability to communicate one's spiritual insights and experiences, making it easier to share one's journey with others. On a deeper psychological level, Turquoise supports the release of fear, doubt, and self-limiting beliefs that may be hindering spiritual growth and self-awareness. This gemstone is a powerful tool for those who seek to cultivate greater self-awareness, spiritual protection, and inner peace, offering clarity, guidance, and the strength to live authentically and in alignment with one's true purpose. As a result, Turquoise helps to cultivate a deep sense of spiritual grounding, protection, and the confidence to navigate life's challenges with wisdom and grace. Its ability to balance spiritual insight with practical wisdom makes Turquoise an invaluable companion for those seeking to integrate their spiritual understanding into everyday life, fostering a harmonious connection between the spiritual and material worlds.

Physically, Turquoise is highly regarded for its ability to support the body's overall health, vitality, and protection. This gemstone has a purifying and strengthening effect on the body, making it particularly useful for conditions associated with immune system deficiencies, respiratory issues, or physical exhaustion. Turquoise has traditionally been used to support the health of the respiratory system, as it is believed to enhance the body's ability to detoxify and to strengthen the lungs and throat. Its purifying properties also extend to the skin, where Turquoise is used to soothe irritated skin, reduce inflammation, and promote a clear and healthy complexion. Turquoise's benefits are not limited to the respiratory and integumentary systems; its protective energy is also effective in safeguarding the body from environmental toxins and negative influences, enhancing the body's natural defenses, and promoting overall physical well-being. Additionally, Turquoise is believed to support the body's ability to regenerate and to recover from illness or injury, making it a valuable tool for those seeking to maintain physical strength and resilience. This gemstone is also thought to balance the body's energy systems, promoting harmony and vitality throughout the physical body. By enhancing the body's natural vitality and promoting balance, Turquoise helps to maintain optimal health and well-being, contributing to a state of physical and energetic equilibrium.

Historically, Turquoise has been revered for its protective and healing qualities, making it one of the most treasured gemstones across various cultures, traditions, and spiritual practices. In ancient Egypt, Turquoise was worn as a protective amulet, believed to bring good fortune and to shield the wearer from harm. Among Native American cultures, Turquoise is considered a sacred stone, used in rituals and ceremonies to connect with the spiritual world and to bring protection and healing. Turquoise has long been associated with the sky and the earth, symbolizing the connection between the spiritual and the physical realms. These attributes are harnessed in modern times to allow individuals to benefit from Turquoise's timeless healing properties. Whether used in meditation, healing rituals, or as part of a daily wellness routine, Turquoise continues to serve as a bridge between ancient traditions and contemporary therapeutic practices, offering a versatile and effective approach to holistic healing and spiritual protection.

Turquoise's unique ability to combine protection, spiritual grounding, and emotional healing makes it an indispensable tool for those seeking to achieve balance and harmony in all aspects of life. Unlike many gemstones that focus on a singular aspect of healing, Turquoise provides a multifaceted approach that addresses the mind, body, and spirit in an integrative manner. Whether used for its mental clarity, emotional support, or physical vitality, Turquoise offers a pathway to a deeper connection with oneself and the world around us. It stands as a testament to the enduring power of gemstones to offer protection and insight, guiding individuals toward a life of peace, wisdom, and spiritual alignment. In an increasingly complex and fast-paced world, where inner peace and protection are invaluable, Turquoise shines as a beacon of strength and serenity, helping those who embrace it to live with greater confidence, spiritual clarity, and a sense of grounded purpose.

Sodalite: A Stone of Truth and Intuition

Sodalite is a gemstone of deep spiritual resonance and intellectual clarity, revered across cultures for its ability to awaken the mind and enhance inner vision. This rich, blue stone, often streaked with white calcite, seamlessly integrates ancient wisdom with a holistic approach to well-being, offering a comprehensive pathway to truth, clarity, and self-expression. As a symbol of rationality, insight, and deep communication, Sodalite embodies the essence of intellectual awakening and inner truth, making it a powerful ally for mental, emotional, psychological, and physical health.

Mentally, Sodalite is celebrated for its ability to bring clarity and order to the mind, helping to enhance rational thought, focus, and intellectual insight. In a world where information overload and mental distractions are common, Sodalite serves as a beacon of clarity that helps to organize thoughts and foster a more structured approach to problem-solving. This gemstone is particularly effective for individuals who struggle with confusion, scattered thoughts, or difficulty concentrating, providing a mental framework that encourages clear thinking and logical analysis. Sodalite helps to dispel mental fog and cognitive dissonance, allowing for sharper focus and the ability to see situations from a balanced and objective perspective. Its calming properties encourage a thoughtful and measured approach to life's challenges, making it easier to make well-informed decisions and to communicate ideas with clarity and confidence. For those engaged in intellectual pursuits, study, or work that requires mental precision, Sodalite serves as a powerful tool for enhancing concentration, memory, and the ability to grasp complex concepts. The structured energy of Sodalite not only clears mental blockages but also aligns the mind with the pursuit of truth and wisdom, empowering individuals to approach life with a sense of intellectual clarity and integrity.

Beyond enhancing clarity, Sodalite is known for its ability to inspire creativity and original thinking. It stimulates the mind to explore new ideas, encouraging innovation and the discovery of novel solutions to problems. For those in creative fields, such as writing, art, or design, Sodalite can serve as a muse, helping to unlock the flow of ideas and bringing a fresh perspective to one's work. The stone's influence extends to verbal communication as well, where it aids in expressing thoughts clearly and effectively, making it an invaluable tool for public speakers, educators, and anyone involved in professions that require articulate and persuasive communication.

Emotionally, Sodalite is known for its ability to stabilize emotions and promote emotional honesty and self-expression. It has traditionally been used to help individuals connect with their true feelings, enabling them to express their emotions in a clear and constructive manner. In times of emotional turmoil, self-doubt, or fear of judgment, Sodalite acts as a grounding force that encourages emotional balance and the courage to speak one's truth. The stabilizing influence of Sodalite helps to calm emotional storms and to bring a sense of peace and equilibrium to the heart. This gemstone is especially beneficial for those who struggle with emotional repression, fear of confrontation, or difficulty in communicating their true feelings. Sodalite encourages emotional openness and self-awareness, empowering individuals to express their emotions with authenticity and clarity. By fostering an environment of emotional honesty and balance, Sodalite promotes healthy emotional expression and a deeper connection with one's inner truth, leading to a more harmonious and fulfilling emotional life.

In addition to fostering emotional balance, Sodalite is a powerful ally in building emotional resilience. It supports the release of deep-seated fears and phobias, helping individuals to overcome emotional blockages that may have been holding them back. Sodalite encourages self-acceptance and confidence, particularly in situations where one may feel vulnerable or insecure. By promoting a healthy self-image and reinforcing self-worth, Sodalite allows individuals to navigate their emotions with greater ease and to approach life's challenges with a calm and composed demeanor. This gemstone also aids in resolving conflicts, both within oneself and with others, by encouraging honest communication and mutual understanding.

Psychologically, Sodalite is revered for its ability to enhance intuition, self-awareness, and spiritual insight. This gemstone is particularly effective for individuals who seek to deepen their understanding of themselves and the world around them or who are on a journey of spiritual growth and self-discovery. Sodalite works by stimulating the third eye and throat chakras, which are closely associated with intuition, insight, and communication. By doing so, Sodalite fosters a strong connection to the inner self and the higher realms, enabling individuals to access their inner wisdom and to perceive the deeper truths of existence. Sodalite also enhances the ability to communicate one's insights and spiritual experiences, making it easier to share one's journey with others and to articulate complex ideas with clarity. On a deeper psychological level, Sodalite supports the release of limiting beliefs, fear, and self-doubt that may be hindering personal growth and self-awareness. This gemstone is a powerful tool for those who seek to cultivate greater self-awareness, spiritual insight, and personal empowerment, offering clarity, guidance, and the courage to live authentically and in alignment with one's true purpose. As a result, Sodalite helps to cultivate a deep sense of inner peace, spiritual wisdom, and the confidence to navigate life's challenges with insight and integrity.

Sodalite's influence extends beyond the individual, fostering a sense of connectedness and unity with the collective consciousness. It is often used in group settings to enhance communication, promote harmony, and encourage a collective pursuit of truth. In spiritual communities, Sodalite is valued for its ability to align group energy, making it easier to work together towards a common goal. It also supports the process of spiritual awakening, helping individuals to integrate their spiritual experiences into their daily lives and to express their spiritual insights with clarity and confidence.

Physically, Sodalite is highly regarded for its ability to support the body's overall health, particularly in areas related to the throat, immune system, and nervous system. This gemstone has a calming and balancing effect on the body, making it particularly useful for conditions associated with stress, anxiety, or tension. Sodalite has traditionally been used to support throat health, alleviate symptoms of throat infections, and enhance vocal clarity. Its calming properties also extend to the nervous system, where Sodalite is used to reduce symptoms of stress-related conditions such as headaches, insomnia, or nervous tension. Sodalite's benefits are not limited to the throat and nervous system; its harmonizing energy is also effective in supporting the immune system, enhancing the body's natural defenses, and promoting overall physical well-being. Additionally, Sodalite is believed to support the body's ability to regulate and balance its energies, contributing to a state of physical and emotional equilibrium. By enhancing the body's natural resilience and promoting balance, Sodalite helps to maintain optimal health and well-being, contributing to a state of physical, emotional, and energetic harmony.

Moreover, Sodalite is thought to aid in the regulation of blood pressure and the prevention of insomnia, making it a valuable tool for those dealing with chronic stress or sleep disorders. It is also said to support the lymphatic system, helping to cleanse the body of toxins and reduce inflammation. The stone's ability to harmonize energy within the body makes it an excellent companion for those undergoing physical rehabilitation or recovering from illness, as it encourages the body's natural healing processes and promotes a sense of overall well-being.

Historically, Sodalite has been revered for its intellectual and spiritual qualities, making it a treasured gemstone across various cultures, traditions, and spiritual practices. In ancient Greece, Sodalite was associated with the goddess of wisdom, Athena, and was believed to enhance intellectual prowess and communication skills. Among Native American cultures, Sodalite was used in spiritual ceremonies to connect with the spiritual world and to gain insights into the mysteries of life. Sodalite has long been associated with the element of air, symbolizing the mind, intellect, and the pursuit of truth. These attributes are harnessed in modern times to allow individuals to benefit from Sodalite's timeless healing properties. Whether used in meditation, healing rituals, or as part of a daily wellness routine, Sodalite continues to serve as a bridge between ancient traditions and contemporary therapeutic practices, offering a versatile and effective approach to holistic healing and intellectual empowerment.

Sodalite's unique ability to blend intellectual clarity, emotional balance, and spiritual insight makes it an invaluable tool for those seeking to achieve harmony and wisdom in all aspects of life. Unlike many gemstones that focus solely on either the mind, body, or spirit, Sodalite provides an integrative approach that addresses the whole being, promoting a sense of balance and alignment. Whether used for its mental clarity, emotional support, or spiritual insight, Sodalite offers a pathway to a deeper understanding of oneself and the world. It stands as a testament to the enduring power of gemstones to foster truth and wisdom, guiding individuals toward a life of intellectual clarity, emotional honesty, and spiritual alignment. In a world where truth and understanding are often elusive, Sodalite shines as a beacon of wisdom and insight, helping those who embrace it to live with greater clarity, integrity, and purpose, creating a life that resonates with truth and inner harmony.

Garnet: A Catalyst for Vitality and Holistic Wellness

Garnet, a gemstone of unparalleled vigor and intensity, has long been esteemed for its potent healing properties and vibrant energy. This captivating stone integrates ancient wisdom with a modern holistic approach to well-being, offering a robust pathway to vitality and balance across all aspects of life. Often associated with the fire element, garnet embodies the essence of passion, strength, and regeneration—making it a powerful ally for enhancing mental, emotional, psychological, and physical health. Garnet's energy is like the steady warmth of a glowing ember, offering a consistent source of strength and renewal that can be harnessed in many areas of life.

Mentally, garnet is celebrated for its ability to stimulate the mind, promoting clarity, focus, and a heightened sense of purpose. In today's demanding world, where mental fatigue, confusion, and lack of motivation are common challenges, garnet serves as an invigorating force. This gemstone is particularly effective for individuals who seek to overcome mental stagnation and procrastination, igniting creativity and fostering a proactive mindset. Garnet's energizing qualities help dispel lethargy and mental blockages, allowing for a more dynamic and assertive approach to life's challenges. It enhances mental acuity, enabling quick decision-making and a clear sense of direction. For those engaged in strategic planning, academic pursuits, or creative endeavors, garnet serves as a powerful tool, enhancing cognitive function and encouraging innovative thinking. The fiery energy of garnet also aids in transforming negative thought patterns, fostering a positive outlook and a renewed sense of determination. Garnet's mental stimulation not only helps in day-to-day tasks but also aids in long-term vision, helping individuals to set and achieve their goals with confidence and clarity.

Emotionally, garnet is renowned for its ability to inspire passion, courage, and a deep sense of commitment. It has traditionally been used to rekindle the flames of love, enhance emotional connections, and build stronger bonds between people, making it a favorite among those seeking to strengthen existing relationships or attract new love. In times of emotional turmoil, garnet acts as a stabilizing presence, helping individuals to navigate intense feelings with confidence and grace. The invigorating energy of garnet empowers individuals to confront and release suppressed emotions, facilitating emotional healing and personal transformation. This gemstone is especially beneficial for those who struggle with feelings of insecurity, emotional instability, or unresolved grief, providing a sense of grounding and emotional resilience. Garnet encourages individuals to embrace their passions, follow their heart's desires, and pursue their ambitions with unwavering commitment. By fostering emotional strength and stability, garnet helps individuals maintain equilibrium during challenging times, promoting a balanced emotional state that contributes to overall well-being. Its ability to stir deep emotional currents makes garnet a powerful ally for those on a journey of emotional healing, helping to transform pain into strength and fear into courage.

Psychologically, garnet is revered for its ability to enhance self-confidence, assertiveness, and personal power. This gemstone is particularly effective for individuals who struggle with self-doubt, low self-esteem, or who find it challenging to stand up for themselves in difficult situations. Garnet works by energizing the root and sacral chakras, which are associated with stability, security, creativity, and sexual energy. By doing so, it fosters a deep sense of self-assurance and empowerment, helping individuals to overcome fears, insecurities, and inhibitions that may hinder their ability to express themselves fully. Garnet also promotes perseverance, courage, and resilience, particularly in situations where one needs to take decisive action, assert their boundaries, or face their fears. On a deeper psychological level, garnet supports the release of old, limiting beliefs, behaviors, and patterns that may be holding individuals back from reaching their full potential. This gemstone is a powerful ally for those on a journey of self-improvement and transformation, offering insight into one's true potential, life purpose, and the path to personal fulfillment. Garnet's energy encourages self-exploration, self-acceptance, and the courage to live authentically, helping individuals to discover their true nature and embrace their unique gifts. As a result, garnet helps cultivate greater self-awareness, self-mastery, and personal empowerment, paving the way for a more authentic, confident, and fulfilling life. It encourages a fearless pursuit of personal growth and transformation, allowing individuals to break free from the past and step into their power.

Physically, garnet is highly regarded for its ability to revitalize the body, support overall health, and promote physical strength and endurance. This gemstone is known for its energizing, regenerating, and detoxifying properties, making it particularly useful for conditions associated with fatigue, low energy, physical depletion, or sluggishness. Garnet has traditionally been used to support circulatory health, enhancing blood flow, oxygenation, and the health of the heart, which is essential for overall vitality. Its stimulating properties also extend to the reproductive system, where it can enhance fertility, balance sexual energy, and promote overall reproductive health and vitality. Garnet's benefits are not limited to specific bodily systems; its invigorating energy is also effective for the skin, where it can improve circulation, support detoxification, reduce the appearance of scars, and promote a healthy, radiant complexion. Additionally, garnet is believed to strengthen the immune system, enhancing the body's natural defenses, promoting swift recovery from illness or injury, and supporting the body's ability to fight off infection. It also plays a crucial role in the detoxification process, aiding in the elimination of toxins from the body and supporting the liver and kidneys in their natural cleansing functions. By supporting the body's vital energy, promoting balance, and enhancing the body's natural healing processes, garnet helps to maintain optimal health, physical well-being, and vitality. Garnet's influence on physical health is not only preventative but also restorative, making it a valuable tool for recovery and regeneration.

Historically, garnet has been revered for its protective, restorative, and energizing qualities, making it a treasured gemstone across various cultures and traditions. In ancient times, garnet was considered a talisman of protection, power, and prosperity, worn by warriors, leaders, and travelers to ensure safety, success, and victory in battle. It was often used as an amulet to ward off negative energies, evil spirits, and physical harm, while also enhancing personal strength, courage, and determination. Garnet's association with the fire element has long symbolized vitality, transformation, and the life force itself, embodying the power to ignite and sustain life's passions and desires. These attributes continue to be harnessed in modern times, allowing individuals to benefit from garnet's timeless healing properties. Whether used in meditation, healing rituals, or as part of a daily wellness routine, garnet continues to serve as a bridge between ancient traditions and contemporary therapeutic practices, offering a versatile, potent, and effective approach to holistic healing. Garnet's legacy as a stone of strength, protection, and passion endures, making it a powerful symbol of life's energy and the eternal drive towards growth and transformation.

Garnet brings the dynamic, revitalizing, and empowering energy of this powerful gemstone into the realm of modern wellness, making it a valuable tool for those seeking to achieve balance, vitality, and holistic well-being. Its ability to stimulate the mind, ignite the passions, enhance self-confidence, and support physical health makes garnet a multifaceted remedy that can be used in a variety of contexts, from everyday wellness to more specific therapeutic needs. As a testament to the enduring power of natural healing, garnet offers a pathway to personal empowerment, transformation, and holistic health, guiding individuals towards a more energized, passionate, and fulfilling life. Whether used as a preventative measure or as part of a broader wellness plan, garnet continues to shine as a beacon of strength, vitality, and healing, offering a timeless source of support, inspiration, and empowerment for those on their journey to well-being. Garnet's influence transcends mere physical health, touching upon the emotional, psychological, and spiritual realms to offer a comprehensive approach to healing and growth, making it an essential component of any holistic wellness practice.

Diamond: A Beacon of Clarity, Strength, and Holistic Wellness

Diamond, the most revered of all gemstones, is celebrated for its unmatched brilliance, hardness, and purity. This extraordinary stone, often regarded as the ultimate symbol of perfection and invincibility, has been cherished for centuries across cultures for its profound healing properties and spiritual significance. Integrating ancient wisdom with modern holistic practices, diamond offers a powerful pathway to clarity, strength, and balance in all aspects of life. As a symbol of the highest aspirations, diamond embodies the essence of light, energy, and resilience, making it an exceptional ally for mental, emotional, psychological, and physical health. Diamonds are often seen as the epitome of perfection and a representation of the divine's purest form, reflecting light in all directions and symbolizing the illumination of the soul.

Mentally, diamond is renowned for its ability to enhance clarity, focus, and intellectual acuity. In a world where distractions and mental fog often cloud our judgment, diamond serves as a beacon of mental clarity, helping individuals cut through confusion and access a deeper level of understanding. This gemstone is particularly effective for those who seek to sharpen their intellect, improve concentration, and achieve mental precision in their daily lives. Diamond's clarity-inducing qualities help to clear the mind of unnecessary thoughts, allowing for a more focused and organized approach to problem-solving, decision-making, and creative thinking. It stimulates the mind, promoting quick thinking, logical reasoning, and the ability to see situations from multiple perspectives. For those engaged in intellectually demanding tasks or facing complex challenges, diamond serves as a powerful tool for enhancing mental sharpness and facilitating breakthrough insights. The high-frequency energy of diamond not only dispels mental blockages but also inspires a sense of mental fortitude and determination, enabling individuals to pursue their goals with unwavering focus and confidence. Additionally, diamond is believed to enhance memory retention and recall, making it an invaluable asset for students, professionals, and anyone who relies on mental agility in their work or daily life.

Emotionally, diamond is revered for its stabilizing and strengthening properties. It is often associated with love, commitment, and emotional resilience, making it a popular choice for those seeking to deepen their emotional connections and fortify their relationships. Diamond has traditionally been used to enhance emotional stability, providing a sense of inner strength and unwavering resolve in the face of emotional challenges. In times of emotional turbulence, diamond acts as a grounding force, helping individuals to navigate their feelings with grace, poise, and self-assurance. The unyielding energy of diamond empowers individuals to confront and release deeply ingrained emotional patterns, facilitating emotional healing and personal growth. This gemstone is particularly beneficial for those who struggle with feelings of insecurity, fear, or emotional vulnerability, offering a sense of protection and emotional fortitude. Diamond encourages emotional resilience, helping individuals to maintain their composure and equilibrium even in the most challenging circumstances. By fostering a sense of inner strength and self-assurance, diamond promotes healthy emotional expression and deepens the connection with one's inner self, leading to a more balanced and fulfilling emotional life. Furthermore, diamond is often seen as a symbol of everlasting love and loyalty, making it an ideal companion for those seeking to strengthen bonds with loved ones or to renew their commitment to personal values and relationships.

Psychologically, diamond is esteemed for its ability to enhance self-discipline, personal power, and spiritual enlightenment. This gemstone is particularly effective for individuals who seek to strengthen their willpower, overcome procrastination, and achieve a higher level of self-mastery. Diamond works by energizing the crown chakra, which is associated with spiritual awareness, enlightenment, and connection to the divine. By doing so, it facilitates the alignment of one's thoughts and actions with their highest intentions, helping individuals to live with integrity, purpose, and authenticity. Diamond also promotes the release of limiting beliefs, behaviors, and attachments that may be holding individuals back from realizing their true potential. On a deeper psychological level, diamond supports the development of inner wisdom, self-awareness, and spiritual insight, offering clarity and perspective on one's life path and soul's purpose. This gemstone is a powerful ally for those on a journey of self-discovery and spiritual growth, providing the clarity and strength needed to navigate the complexities of life with grace and confidence. As a result, diamond helps to cultivate a sense of inner peace, self-empowerment, and spiritual fulfillment, paving the way for a more enlightened and purposeful existence. Moreover, diamond's influence extends to helping individuals break free from destructive habits or patterns, reinforcing their ability to stay true to their goals and aspirations.

Physically, diamond is highly regarded for its ability to support overall health and vitality. Known for its unmatched hardness and durability, diamond symbolizes strength and resilience, qualities that extend to its influence on the physical body. This gemstone has traditionally been used to enhance physical endurance, vitality, and immune function, making it particularly beneficial for those recovering from illness or injury. Diamond's high-frequency energy is believed to promote cellular regeneration and support the body's natural healing processes, aiding in the repair and renewal of tissues and organs. Its invigorating properties also extend to the nervous system, where it can help to alleviate stress, anxiety, and nervous tension, promoting a sense of calm and relaxation. Additionally, diamond is thought to have a purifying effect on the body, aiding in the elimination of toxins and supporting the overall health of the circulatory and respiratory systems. By strengthening the body's vital energy and promoting balance, diamond helps to maintain optimal health, physical well-being, and longevity. Its influence on physical health is both preventative and restorative, making it a valuable tool for maintaining strength and vitality throughout life's challenges. Diamond is also believed to improve metabolism and promote the efficient use of energy in the body, thereby increasing overall stamina and physical performance. Its unique vibrational frequency is said to resonate with the body's energetic systems, enhancing the flow of life force energy (or "chi") and supporting the body's ability to heal itself naturally.

Historically, diamond has been revered for its unparalleled brilliance, purity, and protective qualities, making it a symbol of power, wealth, and spiritual enlightenment across various cultures and traditions. In ancient times, diamond was considered a divine gift, believed to possess the power to ward off evil, protect against harm, and bring success and prosperity to its wearer. It was often used as a talisman or amulet, worn by kings, warriors, and spiritual leaders to invoke divine protection and guidance. Diamond's association with the crown chakra and spiritual enlightenment has long made it a symbol of the highest aspirations, embodying the light of the soul and the purity of divine consciousness. These attributes continue to be harnessed in modern times, allowing individuals to benefit from diamond's timeless healing properties. Whether used in meditation, spiritual practices, or as part of a daily wellness routine, diamond continues to serve as a bridge between the physical and spiritual realms, offering a versatile and effective approach to holistic healing and spiritual growth. The historical use of diamonds in various rituals and ceremonies further underscores their revered status as a stone of purity and divine connection. In many cultures, diamonds were also believed to enhance one's connection to the spiritual world, providing clarity of vision and aiding in the interpretation of dreams and inner guidance.

Diamond brings the radiant, clarifying, and strengthening energy of this extraordinary gemstone into the realm of modern wellness, making it a valuable tool for those seeking to achieve clarity, strength, and holistic well-being. Its ability to enhance mental clarity, stabilize emotions, strengthen personal power, and support physical health makes diamond a multifaceted remedy that can be used in a variety of contexts, from everyday wellness to more specific therapeutic needs. As a testament to the enduring power of natural healing, diamond offers a pathway to personal empowerment, spiritual enlightenment, and holistic health, guiding individuals towards a more radiant, empowered, and fulfilling life. Whether used as a preventative measure or as part of a broader wellness plan, diamond continues to shine as a beacon of clarity, strength, and spiritual light, offering a timeless source of support, inspiration, and empowerment for those on their journey to well-being. Diamond's influence transcends the physical realm, touching upon the emotional, psychological, and spiritual dimensions to offer a comprehensive approach to healing, growth, and transformation, making it an essential component of any holistic wellness practice. The enduring appeal of diamonds lies not only in their physical beauty but also in their profound ability to transform and elevate the human spirit, serving as a constant reminder of the divine potential within each of us.

Clear Quartz: The Master Healer and Amplifier of Energy

Clear quartz, often referred to as the "Master Healer," is one of the most versatile and powerful gemstones known to humankind. Renowned for its remarkable clarity, transparency, and ability to amplify energy, clear quartz has been cherished across cultures for its profound healing properties and spiritual significance. Integrating ancient wisdom with contemporary holistic practices, clear quartz offers a transformative pathway to clarity, balance, and harmony in all aspects of life. As a symbol of purity and infinite potential, clear quartz embodies the essence of light, consciousness, and universal energy, making it an invaluable ally for mental, emotional, psychological, and physical health. Clear quartz is often seen as a conduit for higher wisdom and spiritual awareness, reflecting the light of the universe and acting as a powerful tool for healing and personal growth.

Mentally, clear quartz is celebrated for its ability to enhance clarity, focus, and cognitive function. In a world where distractions and mental clutter can often obscure our thoughts, clear quartz serves as a beacon of mental clarity, helping individuals to cut through confusion and access a higher level of understanding. This gemstone is particularly effective for those who seek to sharpen their intellect, improve memory, and achieve mental precision in their daily lives. Clear quartz's clarity-inducing qualities help to clear the mind of unnecessary thoughts and mental noise, allowing for a more focused and organized approach to problem-solving, decision-making, and creative thinking. It stimulates the mind, promoting quick thinking, logical reasoning, and the ability to see situations from a broad perspective. For those engaged in intellectual pursuits, academic work, or creative endeavors, clear quartz serves as a powerful tool for enhancing mental sharpness and facilitating deep insights. The high-frequency energy of clear quartz not only dispels mental blockages but also amplifies one's intentions, enabling individuals to manifest their goals with greater focus and determination. Additionally, clear quartz is believed to harmonize and align the mind with higher consciousness, making it an invaluable asset for meditation, contemplation, and spiritual practices.

Emotionally, clear quartz is revered for its harmonizing and balancing properties. It is often associated with emotional stability, inner peace, and the ability to process and release negative emotions. Clear quartz has traditionally been used to bring balance to the emotional body, providing a sense of calm and equanimity in the face of life's challenges. In times of emotional turbulence, clear quartz acts as a stabilizing force, helping individuals to navigate their feelings with grace, composure, and self-awareness. The purifying energy of clear quartz empowers individuals to confront and release deeply ingrained emotional patterns, facilitating emotional healing and personal transformation. This gemstone is particularly beneficial for those who struggle with emotional overwhelm, anxiety, or unresolved grief, offering a sense of clarity and emotional fortitude. Clear quartz encourages emotional resilience, helping individuals to maintain their inner balance and harmony even in the most challenging circumstances. By fostering a sense of inner peace and self-assurance, clear quartz promotes healthy emotional expression and deepens the connection with one's true self, leading to a more balanced and fulfilling emotional life. Furthermore, clear quartz is often used to amplify the energy of other stones, making it an essential component in healing rituals and emotional therapies aimed at restoring balance and well-being.

Psychologically, clear quartz is esteemed for its ability to enhance self-awareness, personal growth, and spiritual insight. This gemstone is particularly effective for individuals who seek to deepen their understanding of themselves, overcome limiting beliefs, and achieve a higher level of self-mastery. Clear quartz works by harmonizing all the chakras, but it is particularly aligned with the crown chakra, which is associated with spiritual awareness, enlightenment, and connection to the divine. By doing so, it facilitates the alignment of one's thoughts, emotions, and actions with their highest intentions, helping individuals to live with integrity, purpose, and authenticity. Clear quartz also promotes the release of mental and emotional blockages, offering clarity and perspective on one's life path and soul's purpose. On a deeper psychological level, clear quartz supports the development of inner wisdom, self-awareness, and spiritual growth, providing the clarity and strength needed to navigate the complexities of life with grace and confidence. This gemstone is a powerful ally for those on a journey of self-discovery and spiritual awakening, offering insights into one's true nature and the interconnectedness of all life. As a result, clear quartz helps to cultivate a sense of inner peace, self-empowerment, and spiritual fulfillment, paving the way for a more enlightened and purposeful existence. Moreover, clear quartz is known to amplify positive thought patterns, reinforcing the mind's ability to stay focused on personal goals and aspirations, while also dispelling negativity and self-doubt.

Physically, clear quartz is highly regarded for its ability to support overall health and vitality. Known as the "Master Healer," clear quartz is believed to have a wide range of healing properties, making it one of the most versatile and essential stones in holistic health practices. This gemstone is traditionally used to enhance the body's natural healing processes, strengthen the immune system, and increase overall vitality. Clear quartz's high-frequency energy is thought to promote cellular regeneration, support detoxification, and restore balance to the body's energetic systems. Its purifying properties also extend to the circulatory and nervous systems, where it can help to alleviate stress, reduce inflammation, and promote a sense of calm and relaxation. Additionally, clear quartz is believed to have a harmonizing effect on the body's energy centers, or chakras, helping to remove blockages and enhance the flow of life force energy throughout the body. By amplifying the body's vital energy and promoting balance, clear quartz helps to maintain optimal health, physical well-being, and longevity. Its influence on physical health is both preventative and restorative, making it a valuable tool for maintaining strength and vitality throughout life's challenges. Clear quartz is also believed to enhance the effectiveness of other healing modalities, such as Reiki, acupuncture, and herbal medicine, by amplifying their energy and directing it where it is most needed in the body.

Historically, clear quartz has been revered for its purity, versatility, and powerful healing qualities, making it one of the most widely used gemstones across various cultures and traditions. In ancient times, clear quartz was considered a divine gift, believed to possess the power to connect with higher realms, amplify energy, and bring healing and protection to its wearer. It was often used in rituals, spiritual practices, and healing ceremonies, where it was valued for its ability to clear negative energy, balance the spirit, and enhance spiritual communication. Clear quartz's association with clarity and enlightenment has long made it a symbol of purity, wisdom, and the connection between the physical and spiritual worlds. These attributes continue to be harnessed in modern times, allowing individuals to benefit from clear quartz's timeless healing properties. Whether used in meditation, spiritual practices, or as part of a daily wellness routine, clear quartz continues to serve as a bridge between the physical and spiritual realms, offering a versatile and effective approach to holistic healing and spiritual growth. The historical use of clear quartz in various cultures as a tool for divination, scrying, and spiritual guidance further underscores its revered status as a stone of clarity and divine connection.

Clear quartz brings the purifying, amplifying, and harmonizing energy of this extraordinary gemstone into the realm of modern wellness, making it a valuable tool for those seeking to achieve clarity, balance, and holistic well-being. Its ability to enhance mental clarity, stabilize emotions, strengthen personal power, and support physical health makes clear quartz a multifaceted remedy that can be used in a variety of contexts, from everyday wellness to more specific therapeutic needs. As a testament to the enduring power of natural healing, clear quartz offers a pathway to personal empowerment, spiritual enlightenment, and holistic health, guiding individuals towards a more radiant, balanced, and fulfilling life. Whether used as a preventative measure or as part of a broader wellness plan, clear quartz continues to shine as a beacon of clarity, harmony, and spiritual light, offering a timeless source of support, inspiration, and empowerment for those on their journey to well-being. Clear quartz's influence transcends the physical realm, touching upon the emotional, psychological, and spiritual dimensions to offer a comprehensive approach to healing, growth, and transformation, making it an essential component of any holistic wellness practice. The enduring appeal of clear quartz lies not only in its physical beauty and versatility but also in its profound ability to amplify intentions, elevate consciousness, and foster a deeper connection to the divine and the universe.

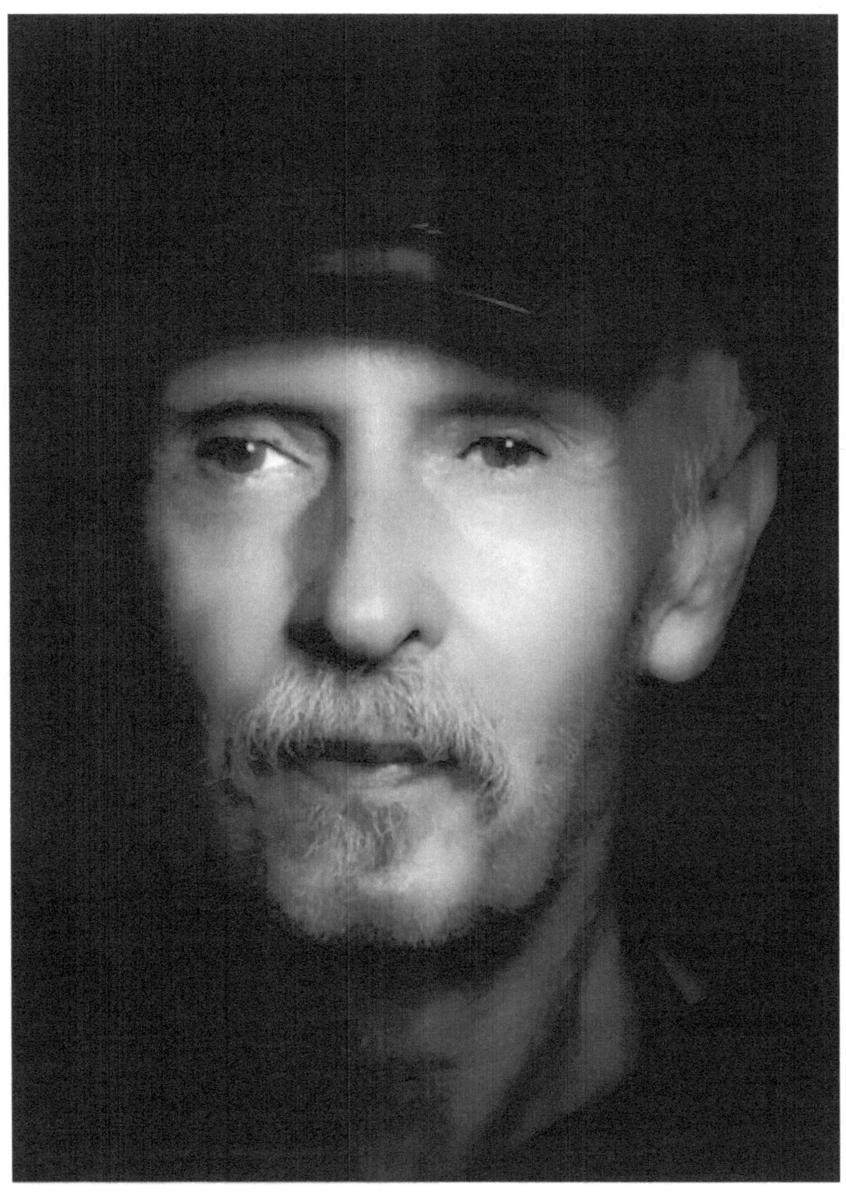

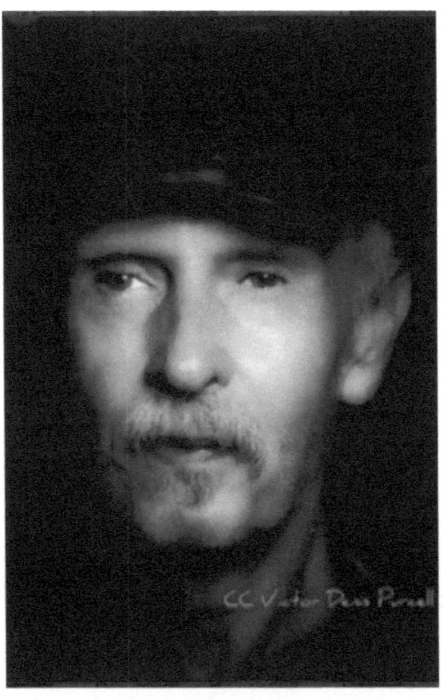

About the Author

Victor Denis Purcell is a certified homeopathic practitioner with a master's degree in educational psychology. With a deep-rooted passion for homeopathic medicine, he has been actively involved in this field since 1982. Over the decades, he has authored numerous books covering a wide range of topics, demonstrating a profound understanding and expertise in homeopathic practices and holistic healing. Through a combination of professional experience and scholarly dedication, Victor Denis Purcell continues to contribute significantly to the advancement and awareness of homeopathic medicine.